Kaye Having Downs Syndrome is Not an Obstacle

1 in every 1.000 babies are born with
Downs Syndrome in the UK each year

Dorothy Hall

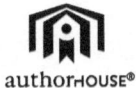

authorHOUSE®

AuthorHouse™ UK Ltd.
500 Avebury Boulevard
Central Milton Keynes, MK9 2BE
www.authorhouse.co.uk
Phone: 08001974150

First published by AuthorHouse 8/5/2008

ISBN: 978-1-4343-7937-5 (e)
ISBN: 978-1-4343-7935-1 (sc)
ISBN: 978-1-4343-7936-8 (hc)

Printed in the United States of America
Bloomington, Indiana

This book is printed on acid-free paper.

Dedication

To my good luck charm, Kaye

This book is dedicated to my beloved Daughter Kaye who stormed into my life 5 o'clock Monday morning on 31st March 1980.

Kaye was not planned, when I found out I was with child, I was worried and excited. I have always loved children and spent much of my time with my niece who was at the time two years old. So being pregnant was sweet expectations, a child of my own.

My waters broke at home and though Kaye was scheduled to arrive on April 4th she decided that it was time to say hello on Monday March 31st

The ambulance was called and I was rushed to the hospital (flashing blue lights to boot).

Kaye exited my life in as dramatic a way as she made her entrance.

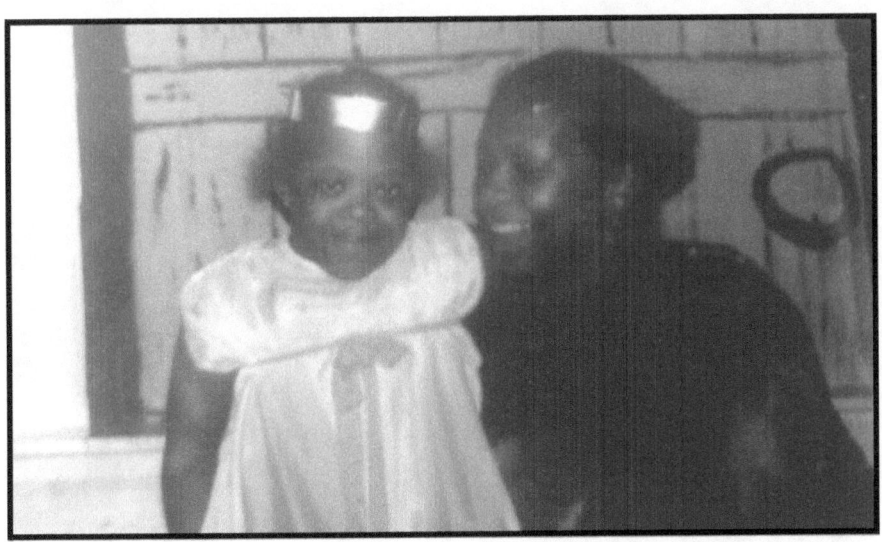

Prologue

The nurse had told us that Kaye had said she was hungry. For us this was a sure sign that Kaye was better.

I was told to prepare at approximately 5:30 pm on 9th February 2007. Though this news was shocking, unexpected and rocked the bottom of my very soul. My thoughts questioned them
'what do they know?' Kaye will be home by the week end.

I was convinced, my faith was strong, and Kaye always come home. I prayed, this was nothing new, only this time, I prayed harder.
Kaye had been hospitalised before. She has had many bouts of serious illnesses in her early years, but in true Kaye style she would shrug it off, get up and say "ooh, I fancy some chips".
I would run to the nearest chippie like crazy because I knew she was better.
This time she did not tell me she was hungry. That was the difference.
The nurse told us what she had said.
What if I was there when she felt hungry?
What did she fancy this time?

What if she had told me, would that have made a difference?

Contents

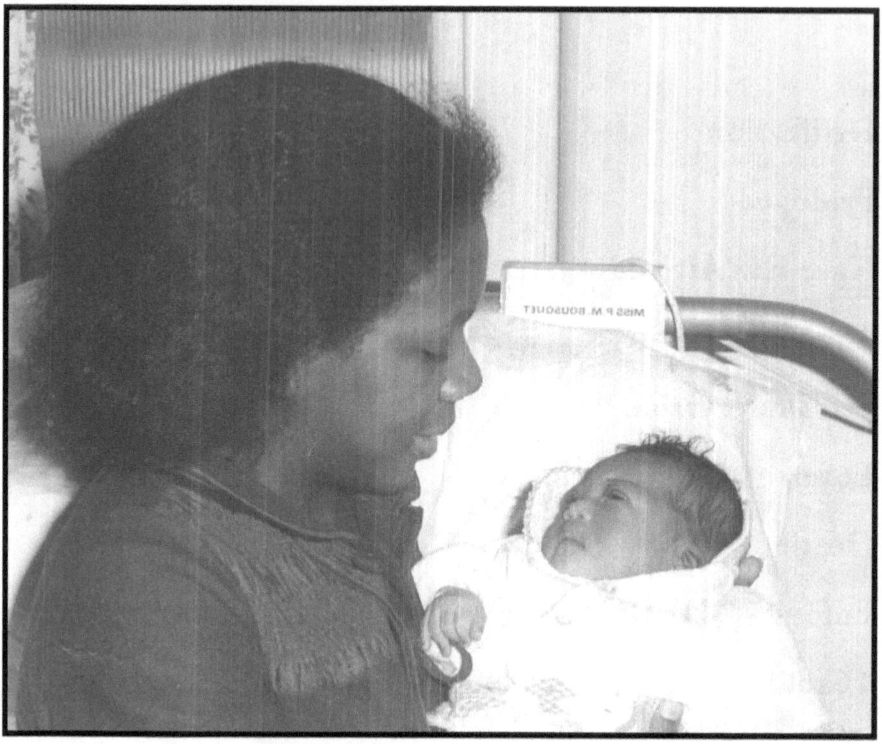

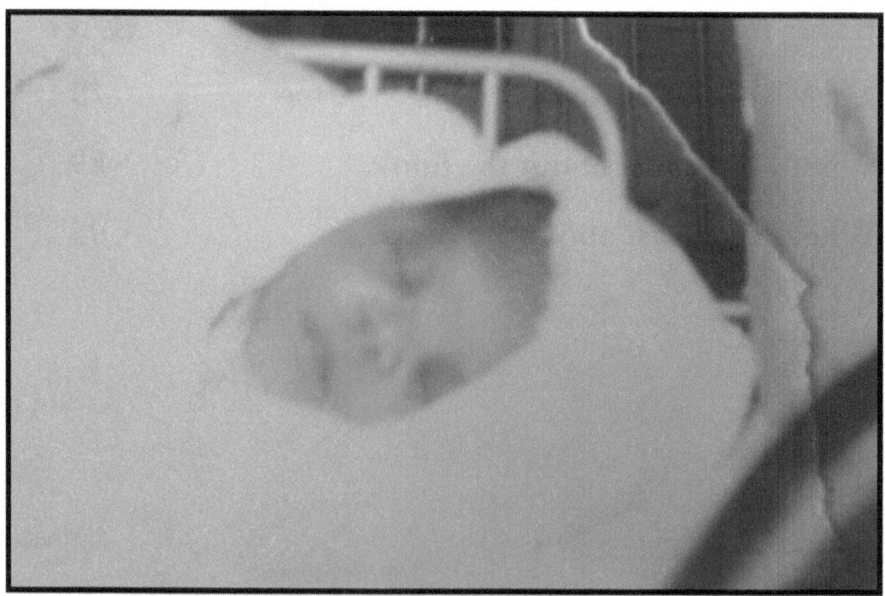

Kaye Has Arrived

I was at my mother in laws home in West Hampstead when my waters broke. I felt for certain that something chronic was happening to me, a hot sensation was running down my leg, and the most excruciating pain in my stomach.
The ambulance came and rushed me to the Mothers hospital in Hackney.

Despite my obvious distress, the medical staff tried to force me to deliver naturally.

"Push, push, you must push", I exhaustingly remember. Nothing happened, nor has it until now. I am exasperated and can push no more.

"Her cervix is too small" came the voice and then through half closed eyes, a mad rush of white coats approached. The cord is wrapped around the baby's neck. We need to do an emergency caesarean.
"What's that" I wanted to ask but was too tired.

Sleep, I need sleep, my eyes closed and open again momentarily.

I have transitorily memories of being told that I would be given an epidural, and what an epidural was. Then a board was planted into my hands for me to sign.

Did I sign it? I really cannot remember. I was fatigued, and frightened.

I woke up some time later that day to be greeted with news of a baby girl.
"She is in the baby unit" the nurse said. "Unfortunately you were given too much epidural and so you are not able to feed her as yet".

I knew something was wrong because I was still extremely sleepy.

My brain computed all that was being said, but I still wanted to see my girl, so they brought her to me.

Kaye was wrapped in a white hospital blanket but she was a beauty.

Arriving at hospital in an ambulance meant that I was ill prepared and not leaving from home meant that I had nothing of my own until a member of my family arrived

My thoughts in my dysfunctional state, half awake, half asleep were that 'this child is mine' not by coincidence then that I was charged with the sole responsibility of raising her from a very early age.

Hospital staff moved us to a private room after Kaye was born. I thought that this was due to the fact that they had over dosed me on the epidural pain killer. To make matters worse, they informed me that Kaye was jaundiced.

I did not complain, I just wanted my girl by my bed side and the doctors promised that they would bring her in that afternoon.

After examining me to establish my ability to look after my baby, Kaye was brought to my bedside. Shortly after, five men in white coats appeared. They took turns to examine my child. I must have been extremely naive, and thought nothing of it. 'Perhaps they were just making sure that the excess drug they had given me had not affected my beautiful daughter. In fact I was delighted that they were conscientious enough to check, to take such care of Kaye.

To me there was no fault with my child, yes she was a little yellow, but surely that was the jaundice.

I sat patiently on my single bed until they had finished and began speaking.

They spoke amongst themselves.

I hated when they do this, it really infuriated me.

"Well?" I questioned, and then the Lead man spoke.

"Can you notice anything wrong with her"?

What a stupid question I thought.

'No' I said impetuously, beginning to think some thing may be wrong. 'Why are there so many of them, and why are they prodding my child?

"What can you see wrong with her?" I asked finally.

This is the science bit

They began to talk about chromosomes using unfamiliar medical language, and when they finally addressed me. The Lead man asked, "Do you understand?" 'Yes' but my heart sank, perhaps something is wrong.

My heart began to race, I sat up straight on my bed I was no longer drowsy. Downs Syndrome? "Yes I know what that is", I had met someone with Downs Syndrome not too long ago, he was such a lovely child.

I looked at my girl, and she was gorgeous, I thought, "this is my girl" and nothing or no one could change that.

My mind was made up, I would do every thing in my power to make things right. I never thought of Kaye as having a disability. I just thought of her as the child I had just given birth to.

They went on, she is Mosaic Downs, (this means that she only has mild not severe learning difficulties) Yet the list of how she would develop (or rather not develop) just rolled off the lead man's lips.

She will not be able to walk until she is five years or so, potty training will be difficult, she may still be wearing nappies right up to school age.

Ah! School, she probably will never be able to read or write to a suitable standard, but there are special schools.

Walking will also be delayed and you might find that her development on the hole will be different from that of other children. She also has a hole in her heart and probably will not live beyond 19/20 years.

'Bastards', I thought (though I did not dear say it) while I listened seething, to the onslaught on this beautiful child I gave birth to only days ago, (bastards).

They were finally finished! 'We shall leave you to take all this in' spurted the lead man.

Take it all in? You bastards, I thought as I got off my bed.

Bent double over my daughter's cot, I really did not know what I was looking for. They had talked about short stubby fingers, small ears, heavy tongue and drooping eyelids, hole in the heart and life expectancy.

But I could not see any of that, she was a baby, she was suppose to have small ears, wasn't she?

Bastards, so what if something was wrong? She is here, and will make sure none of those delays they described would ever impede her quality of life

I began to feel extremely hot and anxious; my stomach was knotted, so this is why they locked me away in this room, away from all those other mothers and their 'normal' babies. I was defiant. In my mind, my child was 'normal' and no one, no one will ever treat her otherwise (after all, what is normal?)

My child is going to be like any other child, better than the average.

The little boy with Downs Syndrome I had met just before Kaye was born stood before me (in my mind of course) and suddenly made me strong, this is going to work, I told myself, we are a team!

I climbed back into bed and just as I pulled the sheets over myself to develop strategies, I saw the white coats appeared outside my door, 'what now' I muttered to myself, but before I knew it the door was open and they were in.

The lead man spoke...
"How are you?"
I looked at him vacantly, Bastard
He continued... "You don't have to keep her you know,"
My heart dropped There are places for children like these Manners forgotten, "Place for children like these?" I screamed

You have gone too far now; I thought, and for the first time in my entire life, now aged twenty something, the foulest words came tumbling out of my mouth "Children like these you...." they were no longer mere bastards.

This went on until my voice faded, and even after they had gone. With my beautiful daughter cradled in my arms, the tears flowed. Quite why I was crying I was not sure, I just knew I needed to cry.

That visit made me more determined, Kaye was going to be the best, and I would see to that. I will protect her from any one and anything no matter what or whom.

I now know how, and our plan was sealed. The need to get my baby home now was more urgent than ever.

The Work Begins

The news had hit me harder than expected I had developed a serious temperature that just would not go therefore I was kept in hospital longer than scheduled . Fortunately, I was able to persuade my midwife that the only reason why my temperature was so high was because my stay in hospital was so stressful and filled with anxiety.

We escaped the hospital on thirteenth April 1980. I was now free to look after my child the way I wanted to.

We returned to my mother's home, where we were blessed to have a warm supporting family who like me saw Kaye as just that, Kaye, a beautiful new baby. There was no mention of her being disabled. Everyone just took it in their stride to support me whilst I supported her.

The midwife called to check on Kaye and me; she made plenty of useful suggestions. One of which was very interesting, in fact it was a question I had for her. "How do I go about getting in touch with people who could support me?" She suggested that I should join a group of mothers who also had children with Downs Syndrome. As you can imagine there were not many people in Hackney in 1980 that had children with Downs Syndrome (or even knew what Downs Syndrome was). Besides who would want to meet with a bunch of people who would sit around feeling sorry for themselves, certainly not me, there were more important needs to address.

I wanted to do something that would help my child to walk, talk, read, write and use the potty on time.

I visited the library a lot and read all I could on Down Syndrome. I bought books, I questioned anyone and everyone I came into contact with who I thought might know....

I was told about a professor Brinkworth who also had a daughter with Downs Syndrome. He was based in Birmingham. I had no idea where Birmingham was, but I knew how to put pen to paper so I did what I knew best. I poured my heart out on paper and soon we were communicating.

Through our conversation, I discovered that professor's Brinkworth's daughter had gained O' Levels. I had similar aspirations for Kaye. I learnt about aromatherapy oils and massages which, not only stimulate the joints but also the mind. This led me to books, articles and seminars, anything that would help me to enhance my learning on how to foster the development of my daughter.

I learnt much from our conversations, and by the time Kaye was two and a half years old she was ready for school.

Forget about the verbal limitations that were imposed on her just after birth. She walked way before her second birthday, she had a good command of language at age two and as for her potty training this went, well I can honestly say that there has never been a day that Kaye was found wet since leaving her nappy days behind at the age of 18 months.

Kaye's first school was The Gate House Private school in Victoria Park Hackney. Kaye started there aged two and a half and left at the age of five. Kaye learnt the rudiments of team work and sharing here amongst other things, but my most precious memory was when we got off the bus to walk the rest of the way to her school.

 Kaye was always quick to get off the bus, (such was her eagerness to get to school) I on the other hand was somewhat slow on that particular day; the driver closed the door leaving part of my coat and my handbag inside the bus.

My daughter went round to the front of the bus,

knocked on the door and shouted "Let my mother out you bastard!"

I would not normally encourage swearing and certainly not from children, but this was different, this is Kaye, aged three and a half years, able to defend herself, and she had my back.

That's my girl I thought, this was the first real sign from her that we really were a team.

No one dared upset me, they would get the same treatment
"you bastard" I wonder where she got that from……..

In 1980 the year Kaye was born Lord Scanlon's Education Act Equal Opportunity for All came into force. Given that she was now five years old I expected her transfer to mainstream school to be fairly straight forward.

Not so, yes my application was accepted but to have

all the practical resources put in place to accommodate Kaye was quite traumatic. I was forced to visit my local MP (Brian Sedgemore, the local education authority Barry Taff was in charge of special needs education at the time) I spent many a hours in his office on numerous occasions. I was even forced to see the then Education secretary Kenneth Clarke at County Hall.

Equal Opportunities for All, my ass, if you were not prepared to force your way in you were not getting in. As the lead man said "There are places for children like these."

Not for my child, she was getting in, one teacher had the cheek to ask me whether kaye suffered from fits and was on medication. Such was the ignorance of the day. So although this Act was in force these people had no idea about our rather special children.

Despite all the initial trauma Kaye settled well here, she made many friends, achieved a prize for reading and was fortunate to have an amazing teacher whom she loved dearly.

Kaye's transfer to Seebright was relatively easy, it just took another visit to Barry Taffe (at Oakway House) to sort out a .3 teacher for Kaye.

Seebright did not share my vision for Kaye and was not as energized about her ability as I was

I was very disappointed with Kaye's treatment at Seebright School. I often turned up at the school to find Kaye playing in the sand pit. At age seven I did not believe that this was appropriate, what made matters worse was kaye had a .3 teacher dedicated to her and she was a fluent reader.

Of course I complained, this gave me the label of an over anxious parent. This label went ahead of me, and did it matter to me? Heck no.

My main purpose was to ensure that Kaye received what was considered to be her God given right and that was for her to be treated fairly and with respect.

Once again Kaye made some good friends in her new School but unfortunately I was forced to move her to a school that recognised her skills and potential.

Kaye moved to a private school in Palmerston Road Haringey, Kaye really excelled here. Like all her other schools her peers were children from all background and abilities, Unlike Seebright Kaye played a full part in the schools curriculum.

At the end of each term the students had a test, with the attention given to Kaye both at home and at school, award winning Kaye never failed to achieve 80% or more in each subject.

Unfortunately the School in Palmerston Road closed as it was being re-located.
Once again Kaye was forced to move School.

By this time she had developed all the social skills she needed to form friendships and to manage herself in a new environment.

I enrolled Kaye into the local special school called Moselle, I was certain that she would be able to cope here. The staff seemed friendly enough on our visit and the location was ideal. It was not a mile from our home so for once Kaye did not have to get out of bed at the crack of dawn. The school also had a bus service which meant that Kaye was collected from and returned to her home at the end of the school day.

I thought Kaye would be as pleased about the bus collecting her from home as I was. On the contrary, she hated it, she wanted to make her own way to school. Kaye had a fantastic sense of direction and could quite easily have done so but me in my wisdom thought it was safer for her to be transported by bus.

Kaye soon got used to the bus rides and her new school. Before long she was not only a bus monitor but also library monitor. She learnt much at Moselle but one of her most treasured skills was learning to travel independently. Kaye just could not wait to get going.

Soon she was making her own way home and even having the responsibility of collecting her younger sister and then her brother too.

Not that Kaye minded any of this, she loved it and was not afraid to point out that she was the big sister and they had to do as they were told.

Kaye unlike some of today's young people never shirked her responsibilities. Yes she was quick to tell you about her rights, but she always accepted her responsibilities just as hastily.

At Moselle Kaye went on many trips, one of her favourites was a trip to Pendarren in Wales.

I remember kaye coming home and raving about walking through dark caves. This was amazing, considering Kaye did not much like walking.

Kaye and her school mates took part in many activities in the community. They sewed seeds and when these were harvested they took part in the young buds display at Alexander Palace. She made any thing from Easter cakes to Christmas decorations.

Kaye's transition from Moselle was easy as there was a link between the college at Muswell Hill and Moselle. Kaye travelled independently to college. It was what she had always wanted, to be able to go on a proper journey independently.

For me it was a nightmare, I could not stand the thought of anyone hurting her. I followed her bus from Turnpike lane to Muswell Hill for over a week. I would leave work early to get to Muswell Hill to follow her bus home too. If Kaye knew this was happening I would have been given a mouthful. Fortunately for me she did not, or maybe she did but just let me off, (I will never know).

Kaye began collecting her siblings from school at age fourteen years old and travelled independently to

Muswell Hill College at age sixteen.

Self Preservation

Kaye's new found freedom was a treat for the entire family, for it was the beginning of some wonderful stories. Kaye would experience some new adventure on her journey every day. We would benefit from her recounting them to us with excitement, on her return. Kaye has seen fights, accidents, people being knocked over, you name it Kaye has seen it.

If you have ever been on a bus with Kaye, you would know of her scrapes with other passengers.
Kaye was taught from a very early age that she was just as valuable as any other human being.
Equality and justice were her daily ration, so when anyone tried to undermine her or interfered with her in any way, her reaction often surprised or caused her

perpetrator to flee rather sharp-ish.

We realised from very early on that Kaye was going to be ok. If you remember, the early nineties was the time when everyone became worried about paedophilia we were encouraged to tell our children not to accept sweets from strangers, not to go off with anyone they did not know and all the usual motherly advice given to children. Of course these rules were drummed into Kaye. So much so that when we took a stroll on a summer's afternoon as Kaye merrily skipped on ahead of us, we were alerted to her by an almighty scream "leave me alone, don't touch me, go away". For a little girl she had a very big voice.

We ran to her where she was standing in front of a well dressed, elderly man it turned out he had said hello to her. The dear man was trembling, curtains were twitching and I was safe in the knowledge that Kaye would never be attacked without being seen and heard.

Apart from the stories Kaye would tell us about her

scrapes on the buses. Friends would also tell us stories of their experiences being on a bus with Kaye

One of these was recounted by a friend, who witnessed a good sized woman sitting down beside Kaye, (and the problem is)? You may well ask.

Well if you knew Kaye you would know she was no sylph her self.

This woman sat next to Kaye and shuffled her into the corner of the seat. She proceed to stretch her rather large arms across Kaye's face and flung the window open.

So astonished was Kaye (or so the story goes) Kaye simply shuffled the woman back to the edge of the seat, looked her good in the eyes, turned and closed the window.

Our friend reported having her heart in her mouth wondering what the woman was going to do. To her surprise and delight, the woman simply sat on the edge of the seat until Kaye got off the bus.

She laughed as she recounted the story, but for me it was quite serious (where do these people get off treating our special children with such contempt)? I knew if she had only asked kaye politely she would have moved up and opened the window. Since she decided to treat Kaye so poorly, Kaye treated her likewise, and I was delighted that she had not forgotten the rules. She is as valued as any one else in the universe.

Kaye made full use of her community resources and was a regular attendee to the local Library, Swimming pool and cinemas.

Kaye loved reading and could always be seen with a book, usually of her favourite star.

Kaye swam like a fish, she loved fun and waves as it meant that when she went down the slides she would be fully submerged in the water and then pop up again like magic.

Kaye kept all the tickets from her visits to the cinema. Once we decided to count up how much Kaye had spent at The cinema. She has spent £350.00 and this was only for half of the year. Kaye thought it was great that she had spent this amount and reminded us that it was her money and her choice so it was fine to spend this amount.

Nothing else was said on the matter, Kaye always won and she was having fun. Kaye loved life and lived it to the full, nothing was too daunting for her, an opportunity came along and she would grab it with both hands. Kaye loved challenges.

Lovers

Kaye had many lovers, most of them she had not met at all.

All the boys from her favourite boy band and her favourite solo male artist (Peter Andre) and of course anyone that she took a liking to who treated her well. Kaye would reciprocate the treatment by looking after them. She defended them jealously, no one could say an ill word against then, nor attempt to come between her and her special friends. Kaye loved everyone and usually forgave the wives and girlfriends when they came on the scene, she would give them the look of scrutiny, but then she would accept them for what they were.

Kaye also had many real loves too; we simply could not keep up with them. Kaye died on February 9th 2007 and on February 13th she received a Valentines card.

It broke my heart to ring the young man and tell him of Kaye's passing. Kaye received many such cards over the last few years. She did far better than I. The only ones I received came from her, her sister and her brother.

It was hard not to love Kaye, she oozed affection, she was funny, kind, loving, and forgiving.

She was a practical joker and as one of her friends puts it, Kaye was a trouble maker.

Death

This is definitely the hardest thing I have ever had to write. You see up to now I have not thought of Kaye as being dead. I used to go into her room every morning to wake her up, say good morning, I still do, at night time I go into her room to say good night and I speak to her on a regular basis.

I visit the cemetery two or three times per week, I do not go there because I think Kaye is there. I go because it's the place where we all gathered on the 1st of march. I go because sometimes I feel a real calling and if I do not go I feel as if I am letting her down.

I cannot believe Kaye has gone; because I was convinced I would bring her home from hospital. I was told the Wednesday before she left us that they would take the tube out of her chest by Friday as she was now doing well. By Thursday all her vital signs were fantastic, all normal. To top it all, the nurse told me that Kaye had said she was hungry. For me this was a sure sign that Kaye was better. In true Kaye style she would go into hospital for something quite serious and after a few days she would come round and say "Oh I fancy some chips" we knew for sure then she was fine and we would take her home soon after. This was how it was supposed to be.

Just before I left on Thursday night I was told that she had picked up a temperature, but I was not particularly bothered by this as Kaye has had very high temperatures in the past and she would shake it off in a day or so. Besides I was jubilant, they were going to take the tube from her lungs on Friday and we would be able to talk again. We had not spoken since she went into Intensive Treatment Unit and I desperately missed our little talk.

I wanted to ask her why she had not called me. Kaye

called me for the simplest thing, if she had had an argument with some one, if she felt unsure or if she grazed herself.

I kept my phone on silent mode but on me even during meetings with clients. If Kaye's name flashed up, I would ask to be excused and take her call, but this day, this day when she truly needed me she never called.

On the Friday Morning before Kaye went into hospital we had spoken before I went to work. She was quite adamant that she would be going to work I could now see signs of her having a cold and I asked her to stay home until I returned to take her to the Doctors. Kaye was insistent "I am going to work". Kaye always won, If I had know that things would have turned out this way I would never have left home.

Her sister and her step father Bob were home with her and I was sure she would go to work.
She never did.

She never told her sister or Bob that she was not well. When they asked she told them both she was fine, why?

On Wednesday 31st January 2007 Kaye told me she was getting a cold, I could see no sign of it but I made an appointment at the Doctors for her any way. The earliest appointment I was told would be Friday 2nd of February. I dropped Kaye to college and all was well.

Thursday 1st February, again all seemed well with Kaye and she made her way into college and returned all seemed well.

Friday 2nd February Kaye showed signs of a cold, I asked her not to go to work but she said she would be going.

I left for work at approximately 8:20 and promised Kaye that I would meet her later to go to the Doctors.

On arriving home from work, Kaye was visibly short of breath, but still lucid. I brushed her hair and she got dressed and met me down stairs. We walked to the car, she had no difficulty doing so.

We arrived at the Doctors but there were no parking outside the surgery.

I dropped Kaye off and she walked into the surgery where she announced her arrival. I parked up and arrived no more than fifteen minutes later.

Kaye was not the same as I had dropped her off only fifteen minutes ago.

I had to insist that she was seen now and not in five minutes time when our appointment was due.

Kaye was admitted to hospital on the 2nd February at 5:00 pm by 10:00 pm she was feeling much better and we were able to communicate again. She said she was thirsty, I fed her with water, she said she did not want the oxygen mask on her face. She has never liked it, she has had to use it on many occasions. I asked whether there was another option. I was told she could have a tube in her throat but that she would be sedated. I explained it to Kaye and we agreed. I stayed with her until she fell asleep. I arrived home at approximately 1:00 am, I called the hospital at approximately 3:00 am to find out whether they had made Kaye more comfortable (she hated that mask on her face and I was worried it may be irritating her eyes).

On the morning of Saturday 3rd February I arrived at Hospital and the tube was in. I was no longer able to speak to my baby.

I laid at her feet and caressed them.

Sunday the 4th February, I talked to her telling her all that was happening at home, and laid at her feet until it was time to go.

Monday the 5th February was much the same.

By Tuesday 6th February Kaye's vital signs were looking better on the monitor.

On Wednesday 7th February, the sedation was reduced, I was told that Kaye was doing well and that the tube would be removed by Friday 9th February. I was also told that Kaye had said she was hungry.
This was a good sign.

Thursday 8th February I looked on her Monitor and it was perfect, all her vital signs were normal. I had brought in her own night clothes and clothes to go home in they waited in the boot of my car. I brought in her MP3 Player and head phones so that she could listen to her music.

Though the doctors had told me that she had picked up a temperature, I went home jubilant. Kaye always shook off those temperatures.

Friday 9th February, I arrived at the Hospital, took one look at her monitor and knew something was wrong.

I was told the temperature had gotten worse and that none of the antibiotics were working. They had tried many and were still trying.

The idea of death was never in my thoughts, I was not unduly worried, I really believed that I would bring Kaye home at the weekend.

At about 3:00 pm I was told that the consultant wanted to speak to me, I did wonder what that was about, but again I was not that really worried, I remained strong, my faith was strong.

I was not seen by the consultant until 5.00 pm that evening when I was told to prepare for my daughters death. "We are going round in circles" I was told, "None of the antibiotics are working".

For the first time my stomach knotted, but still my faith was strong and I thought 'what do they know'.

I prayed harder and harder. I rang certain people,

people Kaye would have wanted to see, but not her brother and sister. I was sure I was taking her home to see them.

Nonetheless her sister came and as she spoke to Kaye her heart rate (which was now racing) went down a little.

After Kaye's sister had left, Kaye's sister's god mother, Kaye's god mother and I took turns to speak to Kaye. Her heart rate fluctuated and at approximately 12 Midnight Kaye flashed us a smile, her face was calm and beautiful and she was gone.

On Friday 2nd February I took Kaye to the Doctors as planned. On seeing Kaye our doctor called the ambulance, Kaye was put on a bed and wheeled into the ambulance and I got in with her. It took off, flashing blue light to boot.

Kaye never walked back in our home with me. She left me on 9th February 2007; she left me with a smile.

I know something sinister happened in that Hospital otherwise Kaye would be here today.

I know my daughter did not just go.

They denied me the privilege of seeing my dead child from the 9th to 14th February. I was told at the time of death she would need to have an autopsy so I could not touch her. I rang up every day after her death, but I was told I could not see her. On the 14th February I called the hospital again to confirm that she had had the autopsy, I was told she did not need one, then why did she die? I asked as I cried.

Eulogy – MY BIG SIS 'Kaye'

<u>Think Big</u>

Kaye began her education at Gate House private school in Hackney, where she stayed until she was five years old. Kaye learned much at Gate house but mother was determined that Kaye would attend main stream school, so Kaye was moved to Queensbridge Infant School where she would develop the skills to interact with people from all walks of life. Kaye progressed here and was reading fluently by the time she had left. She moved to Seebright Primary School, and made many friends here however mother was not content with the teaching or treatment of Kaye (she had great aspirations for Kaye) so she was moved to Palmerston Independent Christian School in Haringey. Kaye excelled here and achieved no less than 80% in her end of term tests in English, Maths and Social Science.

Kaye had now grasped all the skills of operating in a so called "normal world" so mother moved her to Moselle School where she learnt new skills and developed those she had already possessed. Kaye learnt much at Moselle and became a library monitor, a register monitor; she was also responsible for helping the younger children in the blue class.

One of Kaye's most enjoyable moments was learning to travel independently. She simply could not wait to get going, she hated the bus coming to collect her, though she liked the job of bus monitor.

Kaye moved from the lower school to the upper school, she then moved to Muswell Hill College, by this time Kaye was an independent traveller and was in her element. The independence was like a new lease of life, and when she was given the responsibility of collecting Christian and I, she excelled at it; she really took charge of us and made sure we were guided safely home.

At Muswell Hill College two of Kaye's preferred subjects were Horticulture and Performing Arts for which she achieved pass certificates. The Muswell Hill site was closed and Kaye transferred to The College of North East London where she, again made many friends and was awarded credits towards NVQ level 1 in Hairdressing as well as a City and Guilds certificate in cookery to name but a few. Despite the new college being a lot closer than the one in Muswell Hill, Kaye use to leave home at the same time. So correct me if I'm wrong but I doubt she was ever late.

<u>Think inside</u>

Kaye was the perfect blue print for a human being. She was kind, compassionate, loving, forgiving, resilient, hard working, punctual and fair. Kaye did not take any nonsense from anyone, no matter who they were or where she was. If you have ever been on the bus with Kaye you will know exactly what I'm talking about. She could cut you down with a look and pick you up with a smile moments after. Kaye would never hold a grudge.

Kaye was our big sister and she played her role perfectly. A better big sister no one could have wanted.

To us Kaye did not have a disability, she did not have a heart condition or any thing else, she was just our big sister. She collected and walked us home from school. She cooked for us, she chastised and disciplined us, and she brought us presents. She locked us out of her room when she wanted us to stay out and let us in when she wanted us to come in.

Kaye and I shared a room for a while and although Kaye liked her space. Whenever I was afraid or upset she would always put an extra pillow on her bed for me to sleep next to her.

Kaye was always there whenever any of us was sick; she use to sit next to us and rested our heads on her lap, then ask if we were going to have a wash sometime today. Kaye was our big sister in every sense of the word.

Think small

Kaye hated rice and peas and always picked out all the peas, and would either leave them in the pot so there was almost more peas than rice for us to eat or leave them on the side of her plate. Another great hate was having blood test which she had many.

Think Happy

Kaye loved life and she lived it to the full, there was no stopping her. She was always out with friends, in the café, at the pictures and down the pub, drinking a pint of Stella. Her friends were very special to her and she had many. Kaye loved music from all genres; when she came home with albums by people like Take That, Peter Andre and Boy Zone we would ask her where she was going with that rubbish. And I swear she used to play the music loud on purpose just to educate us or punish us for bad mouthing her purchase. Other times she would play some tunes which would make me go into her room to dance with her. But she would always stop dancing, and put her hand on her chin, look at me and smile as if to say "you know I'm a connoisseur".

Kaye was a fantastic story teller and always kept us entertained by her weird and wonderful experiences. A day out for Kaye was like a whole week's expedition as we knew that she would return with some wondrous tails of what she had experienced. If you never heard any stories about the birds and her chips or about the fires, flights or hit and runs down Wood Green (which for some reason she would always see) you missed out.

Our world will never be the same again, it has fallen apart and quite frankly our holidays and home videos will never be the same again.

But over the last few weeks we have come to realised that Kaye was put on earth for a purpose and she has executed that job with precision, and now she must return to her maker and to Junior our other brother. It is now his turn to be with this special sister.

Kaye has taught the world that there is no disability apart from the restrictions that you put on yourselves.

We love you Kaye
Thank you for bringing such richness to our lives
And thank you Jesus for putting her in our family

At the dentist

I had a tooth ache on Saturday

so my mother says, off to the dentist

you must go on Monday.

I like the chair, because it goes up

and down,

but I don't like the dentist to mess

around. .

He puts some music in my ear,

then he speaks to mother so 1 can't

hear.

My mother agrees, what she agrees I

don't care.

I don't like the dentist, but I do like

this chair.

For Kaye,

Dorothy A Hall

Poets Corner is your chance to get in
to print. Send your unpublished poems to
Poets Corner, The Voice, 370 Cold Harbour

Lane, London SW9 8PL.

Kaye Danielle - Tribute delivered by Patricia Hall at
the funeral service in High Cross United Reformed

Church on 1 March 2007

Introduction

Kaye was my niece, a very special niece with whom I formed a bond from the day she was born. She was my sister's daughter.

Kaye was loving, kind and thoughtful, with a tremendous sense of humour. She would laugh at herself as well as others and was never easily offended. She loved to play practical jokes on her siblings, Christian and Mickela.

She was always well prepared. She would buy cards for special occasions well in advance and never forgot a birthday. The last example of this was the birthday card she bought for Mickela whose birthday was several days after Kaye's passing.

Kaye and her mother had a symbiotic relationship. In

an uncanny sort of way kaye's birth gave her mother strength to overcome all sorts of obstacles and together they went on to achieve great things when others would have given up.

High Achiever

Kaye was a high achiever, she had determination, drive and a mother who made sure that her ambitions were not thwarted by anyone who sought to take advantage of her.

Kaye did not allow her disability to hold her back. She went on to college and out to work in the big wide world. Nothing pleased her more than to pick up her salary.

She was always prepared to try different things. She went on all the rides at Alton Towers and motor biking in Tunisia, where she spent her last holiday with her family in December.

Her biggest passions were music, swimming and the cinema.

Kaye spent most of her money on CD's and magazines. If she had gone on to Mastermind her specialist subject would have been POP music with special focus on Peter Andre.

Kaye swam like a fish. She was not content with splashing around and causing a disturbance in the water. Unlike me who is afraid to get my face and hair wet – she preferred swimming fully submerged. With a little more time and preparation she could have gone on to win gold for Jamaica in the 2012 Olympics. That was our Kaye.

Kaye spent many memorable weekends with me and my family. Her knock on at the door was distinctive. She was always the first to arrive at the door. Even without seeing her, we knew who was there. We would lock in a tight embrace. Her warmth was overwhelming.

Thanks
Thanks to my wonderful friends
and family for always being there
for us and for proof reading our
Kaye's book

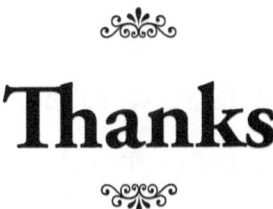

Thanks

Special thank you:

To our lord, for putting our Kaye in our lives for nay– on twenty seven wonderful years.

Thank you Kaye, for making our lives so much richer for having you. We know not what we will do now but we know that you will continue to be with us and guide us.

We will remember you fondly and will live by the standards you have set for us. These will make us laugh, cry, sad, and happy, but knowing that you are always in our hearts should keep us sane.

To the First Step Trust for providing Kaye with her first real work experience

To College of North East London for providing a safe place that Kaye truly loved.

To Moselle School, for Supporting Kaye with her independent travel.

When I was told to prepare my heart sank, I felt an emptiness that I tried to fill with my tears. I wept and I cried but still I believed.

We had a plan, you and I that we would leave

Your home coming clothes still lay in the boot of my car and your coat by the door while I waited for the call.

I held your hand, my baby, till you went cold, but I still did not believe that you had closed the door.

We had a plan, you and I that we would leave.
My faith was strong and I believed,
I believed, I believed, I believed.

I took it for granted that our plans were God's plan, but now I find that my faith was not that strong

I was always guided by you my, sweet. I pray that you will keep me strong.

Our hearts will always be bounded together my baby, and I know that is GOD'S PLAN

LOVE MUM

Photos

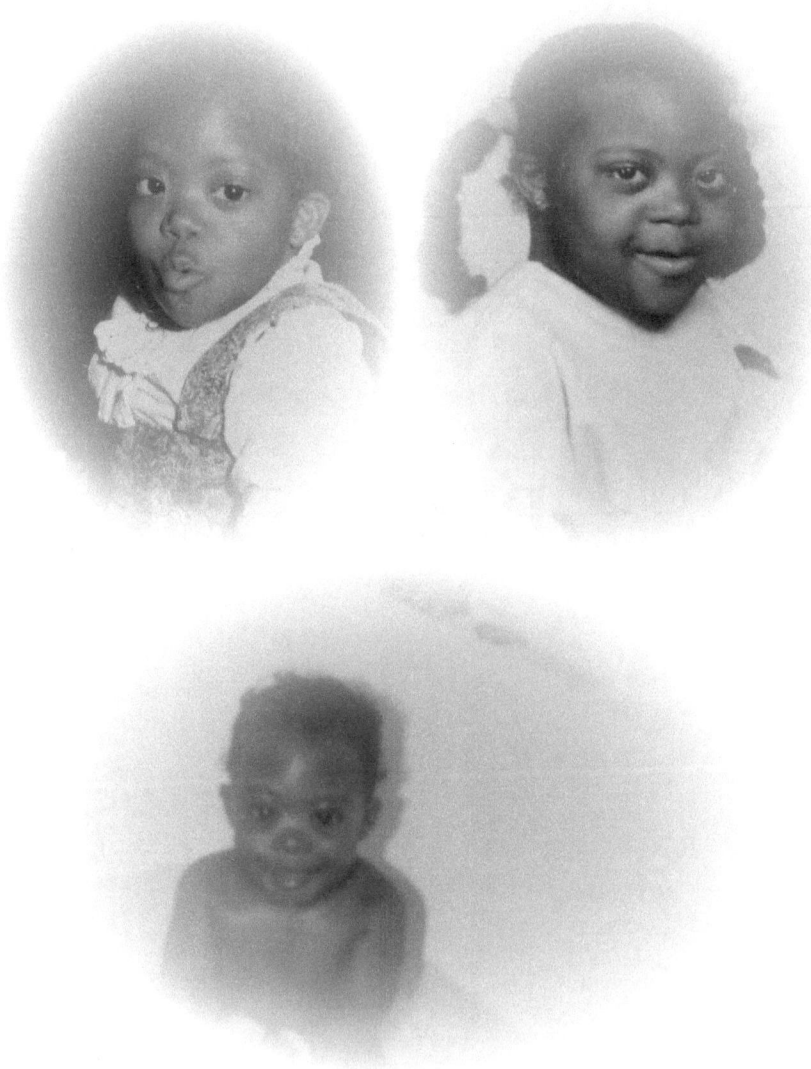

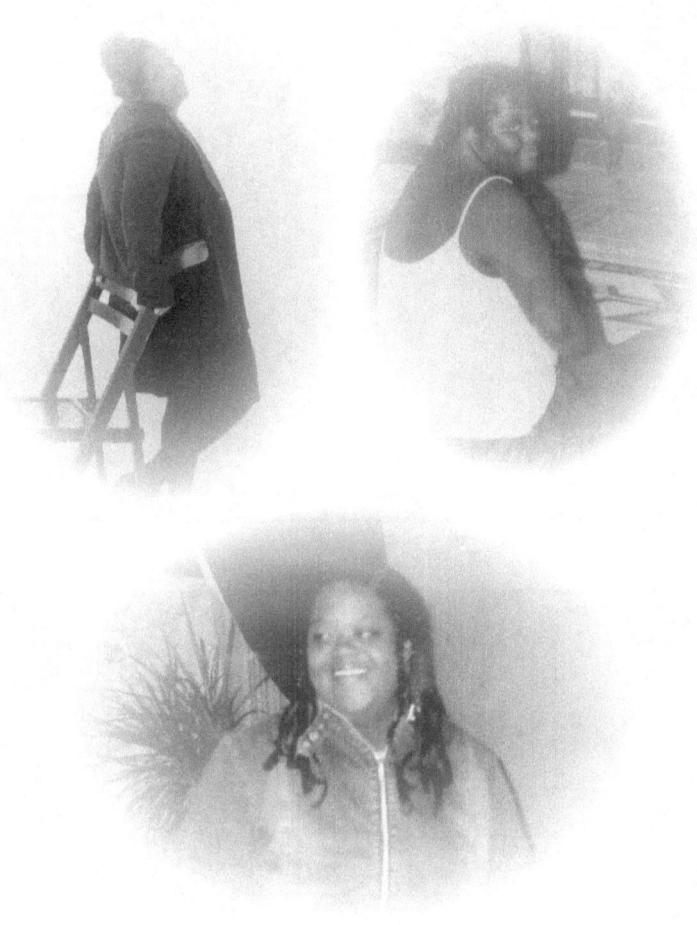

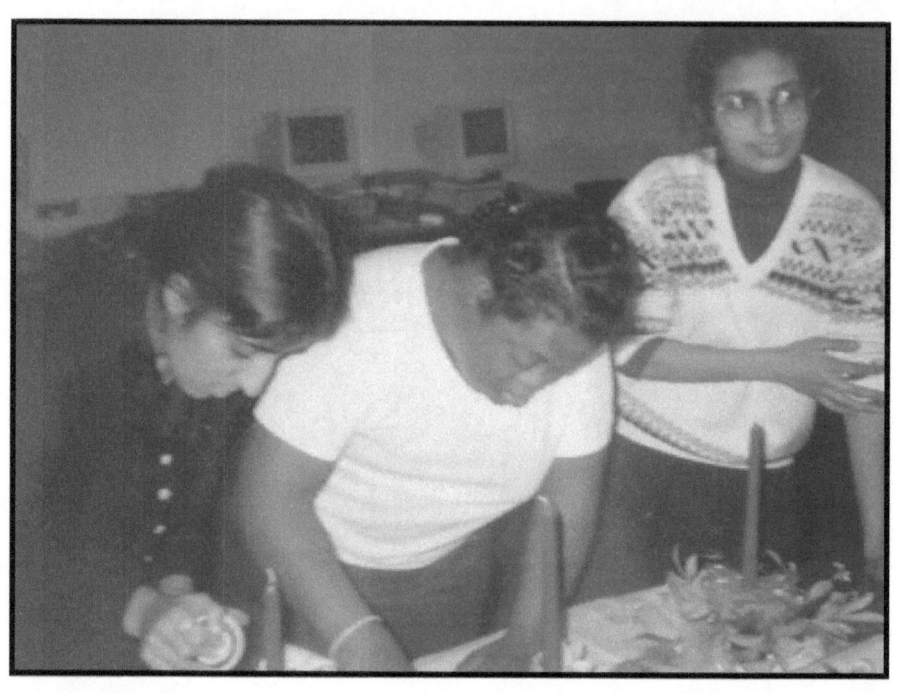

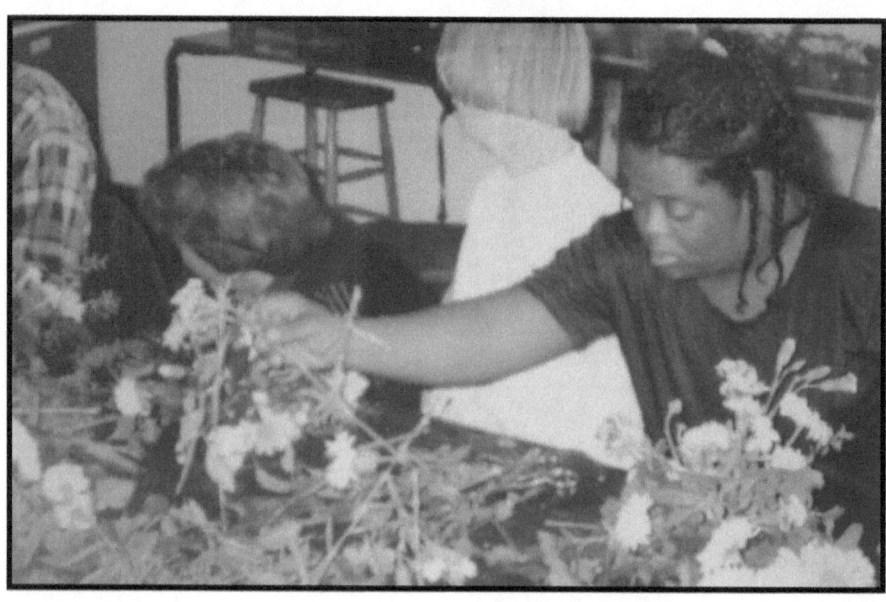

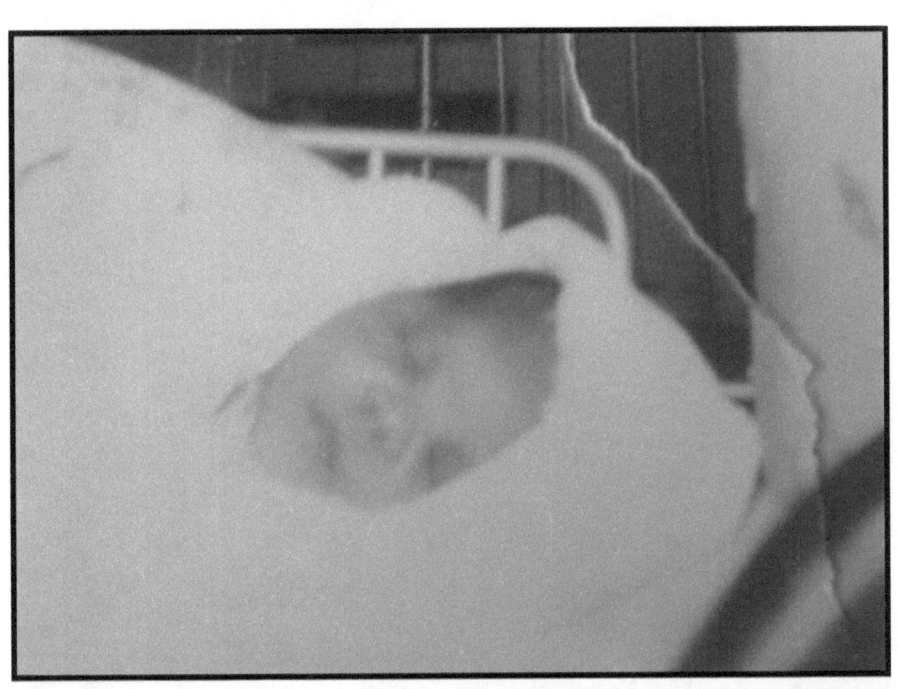

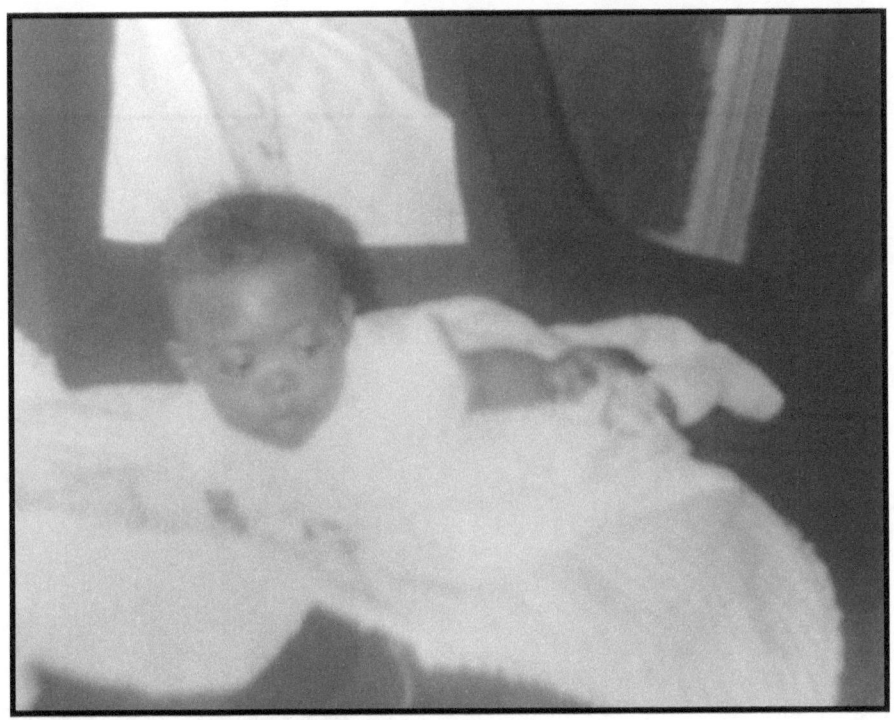

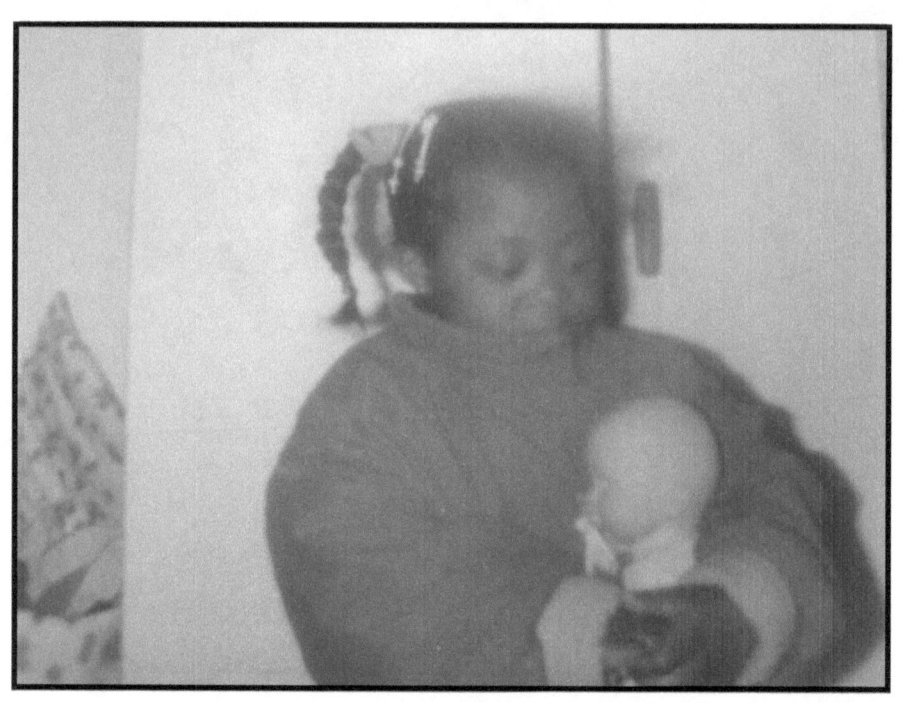

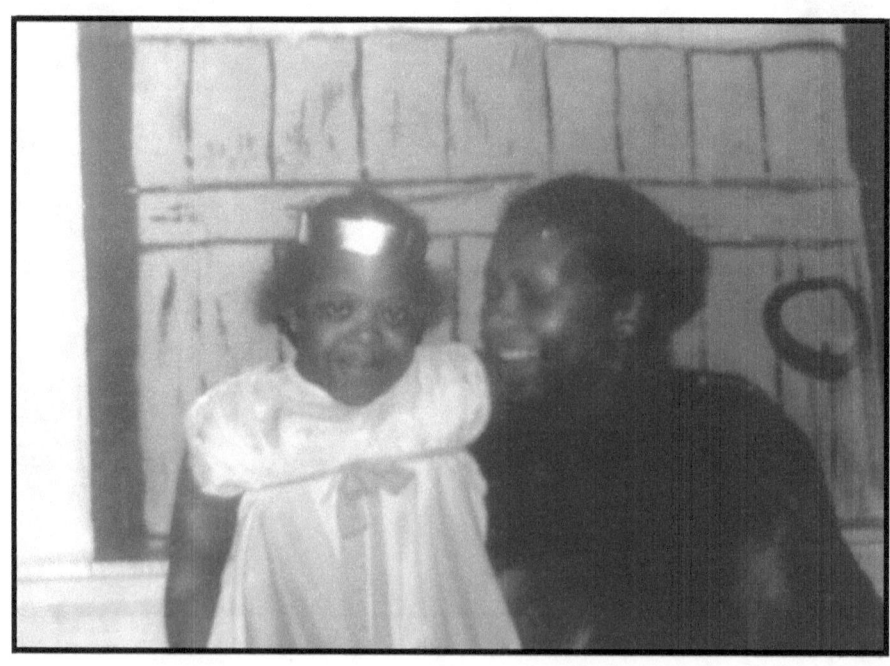

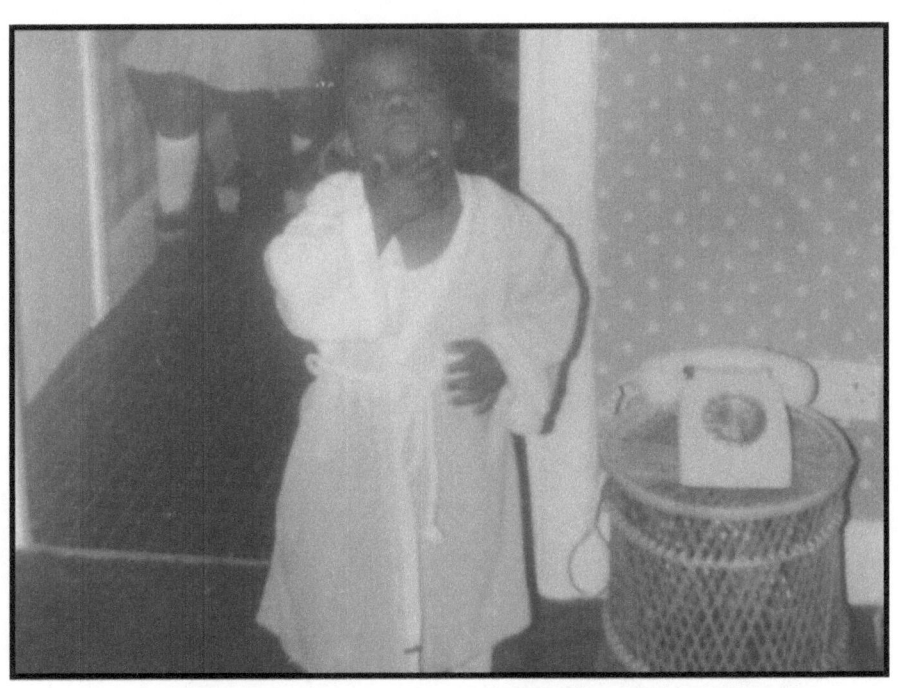

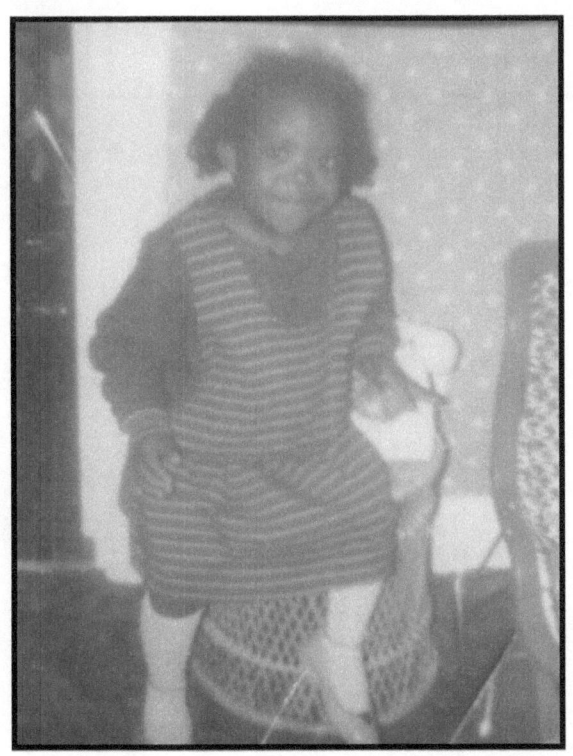

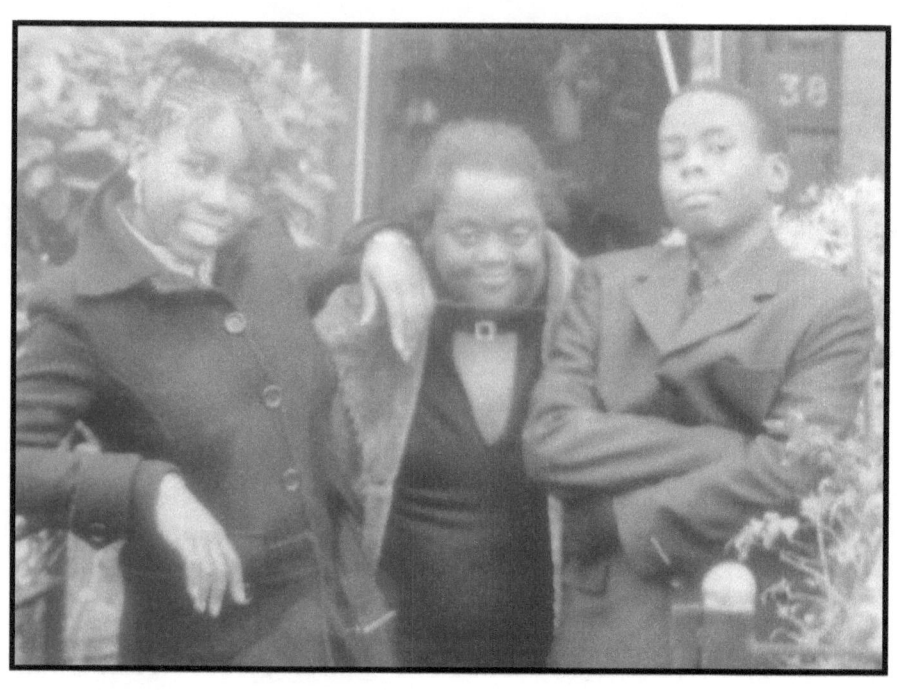

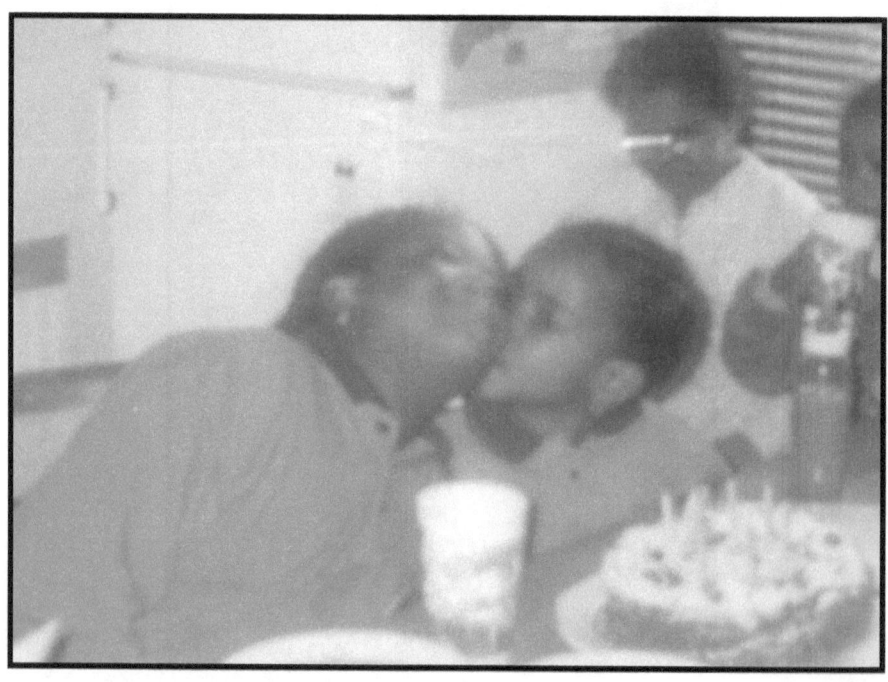

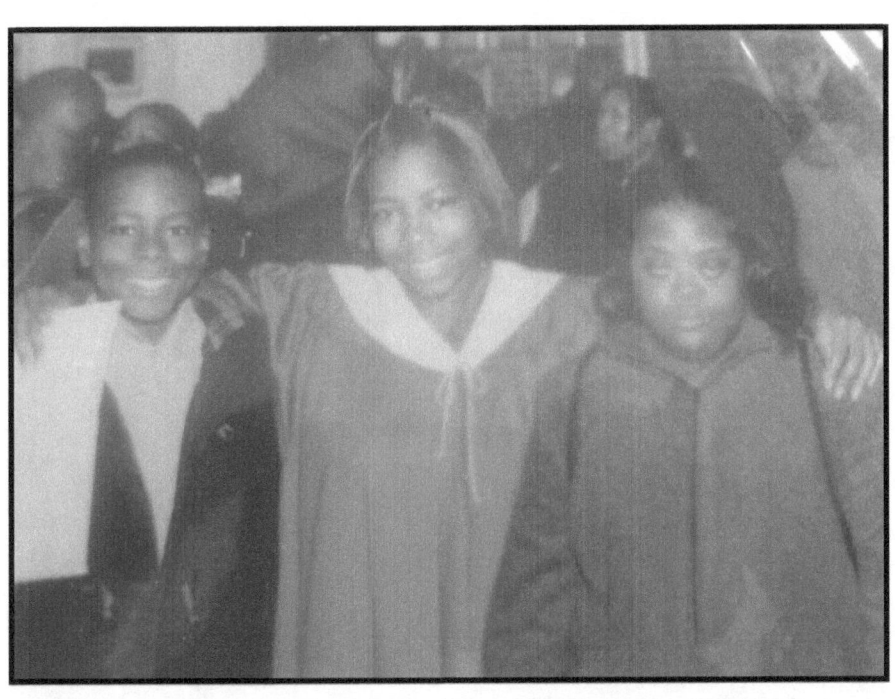

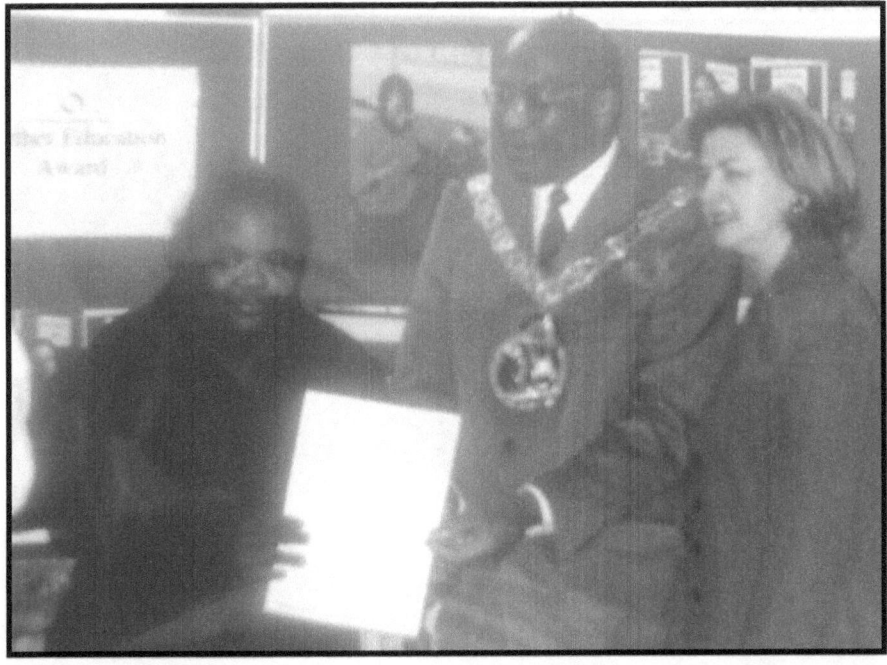

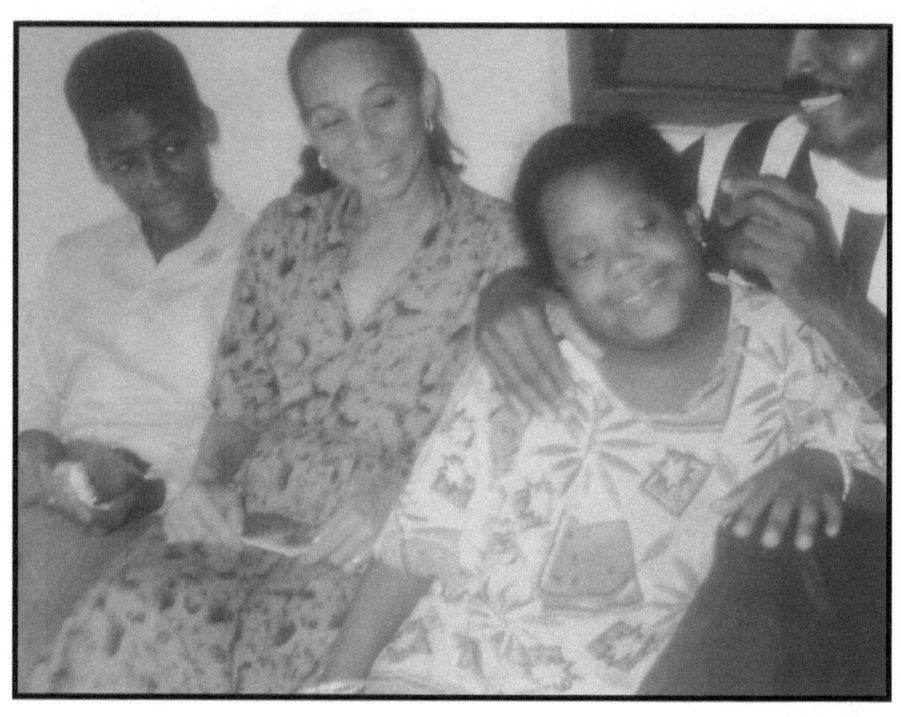

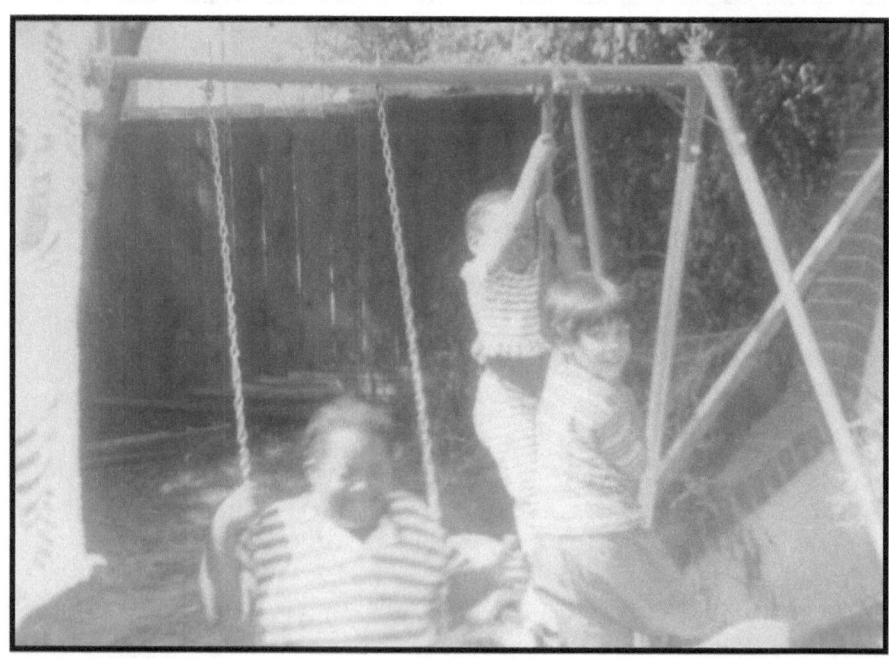

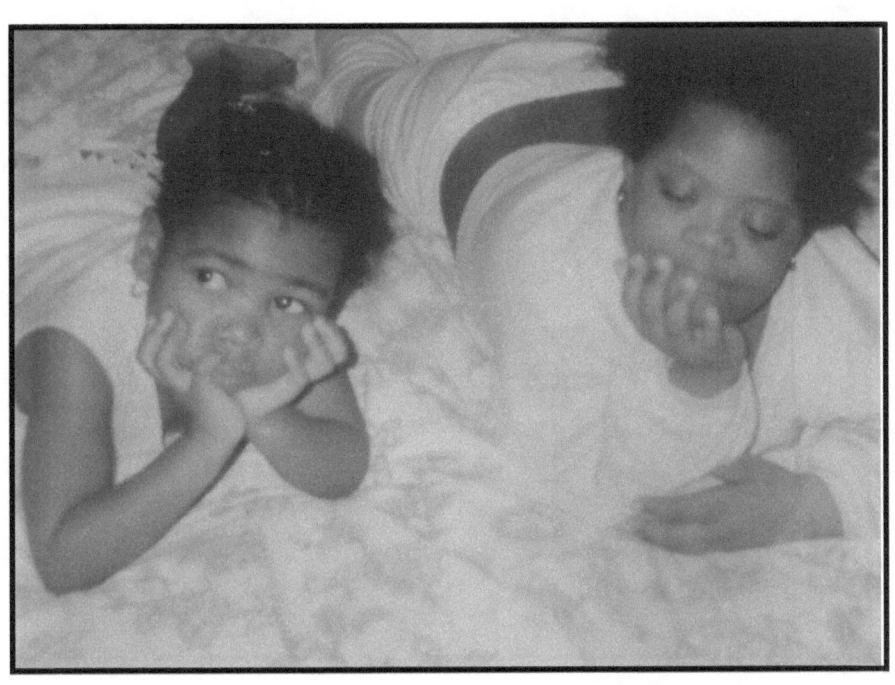

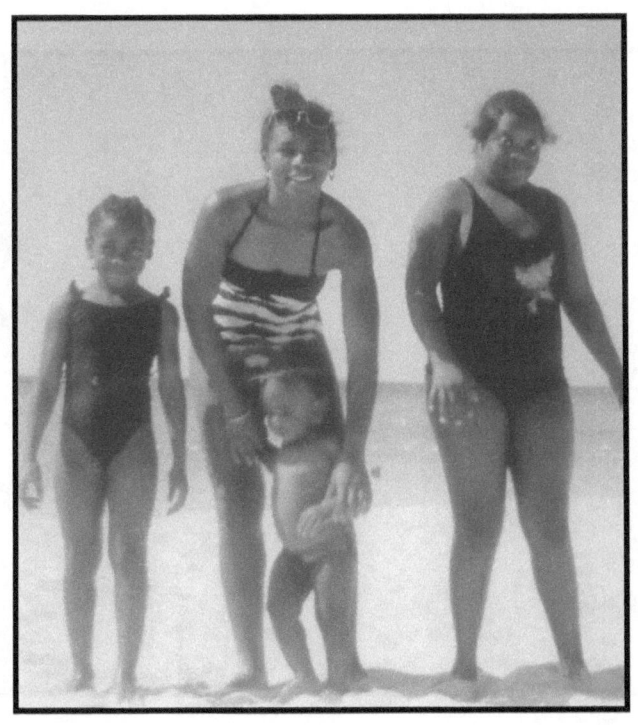

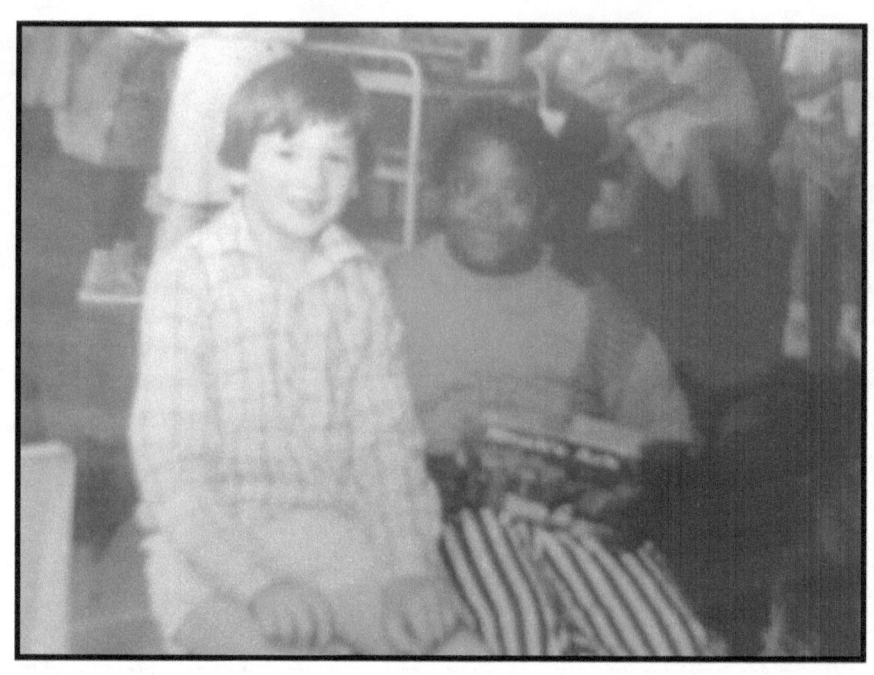

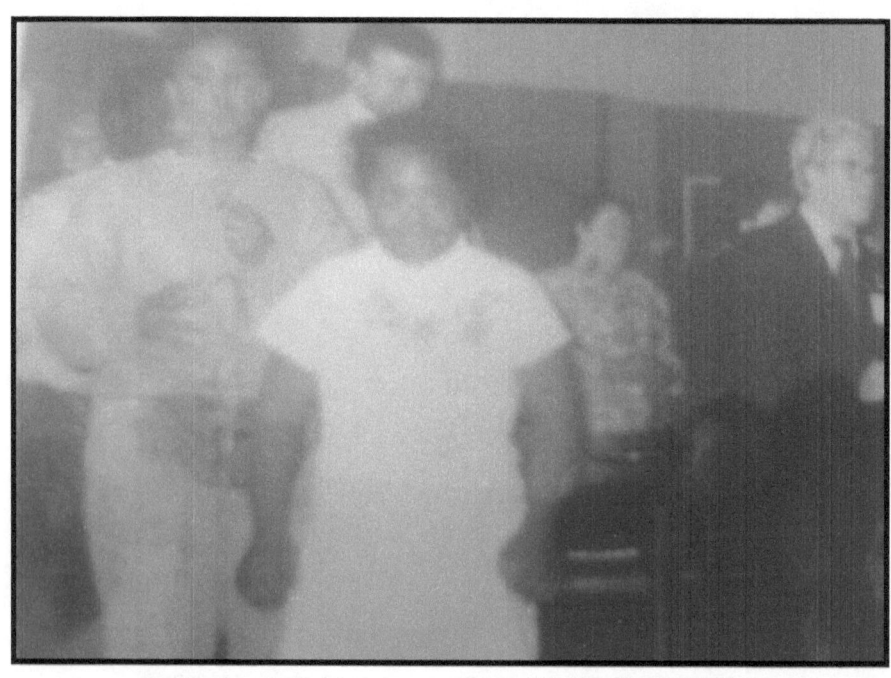

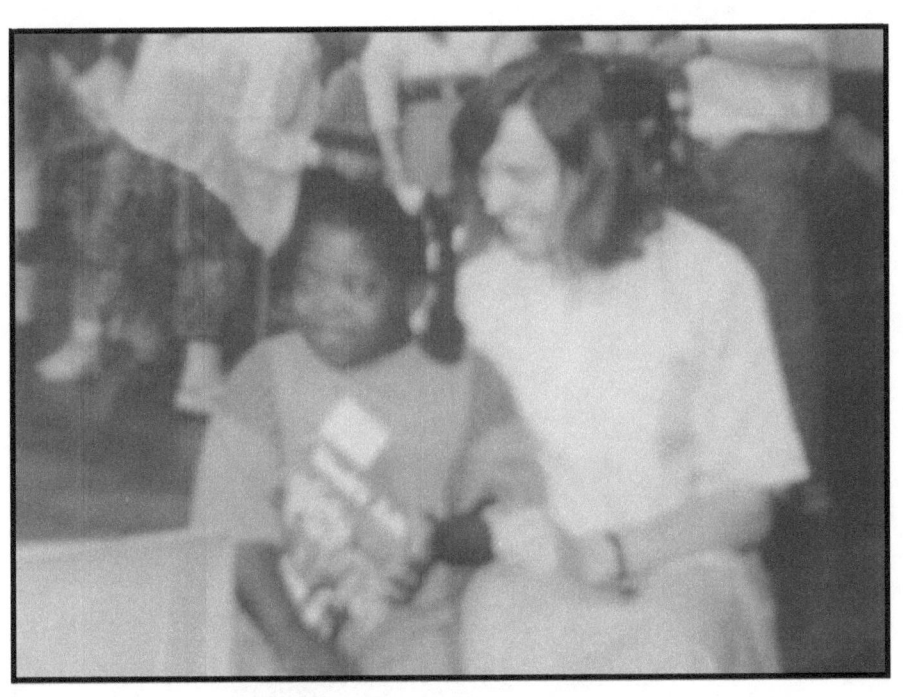

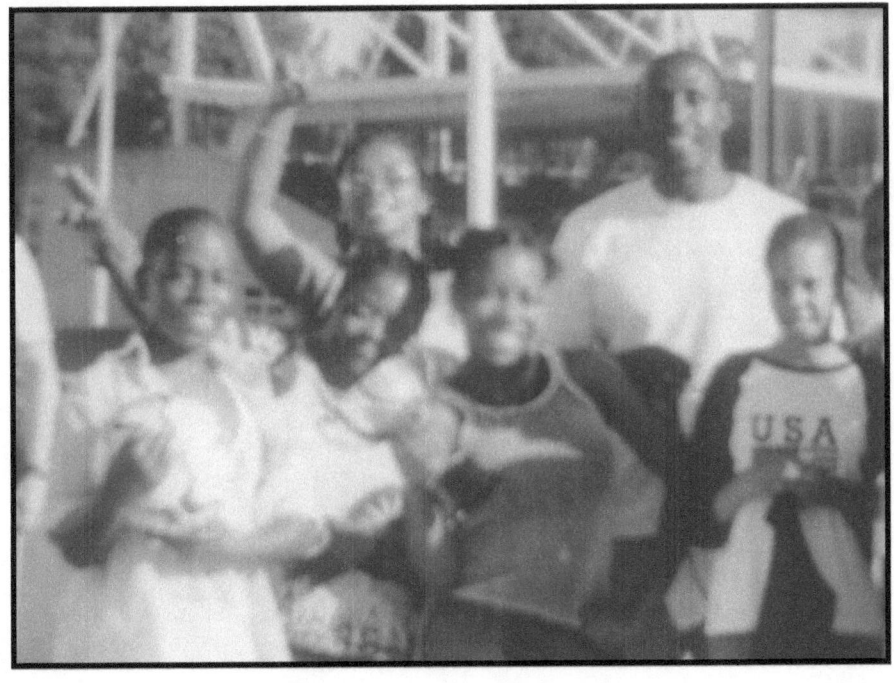

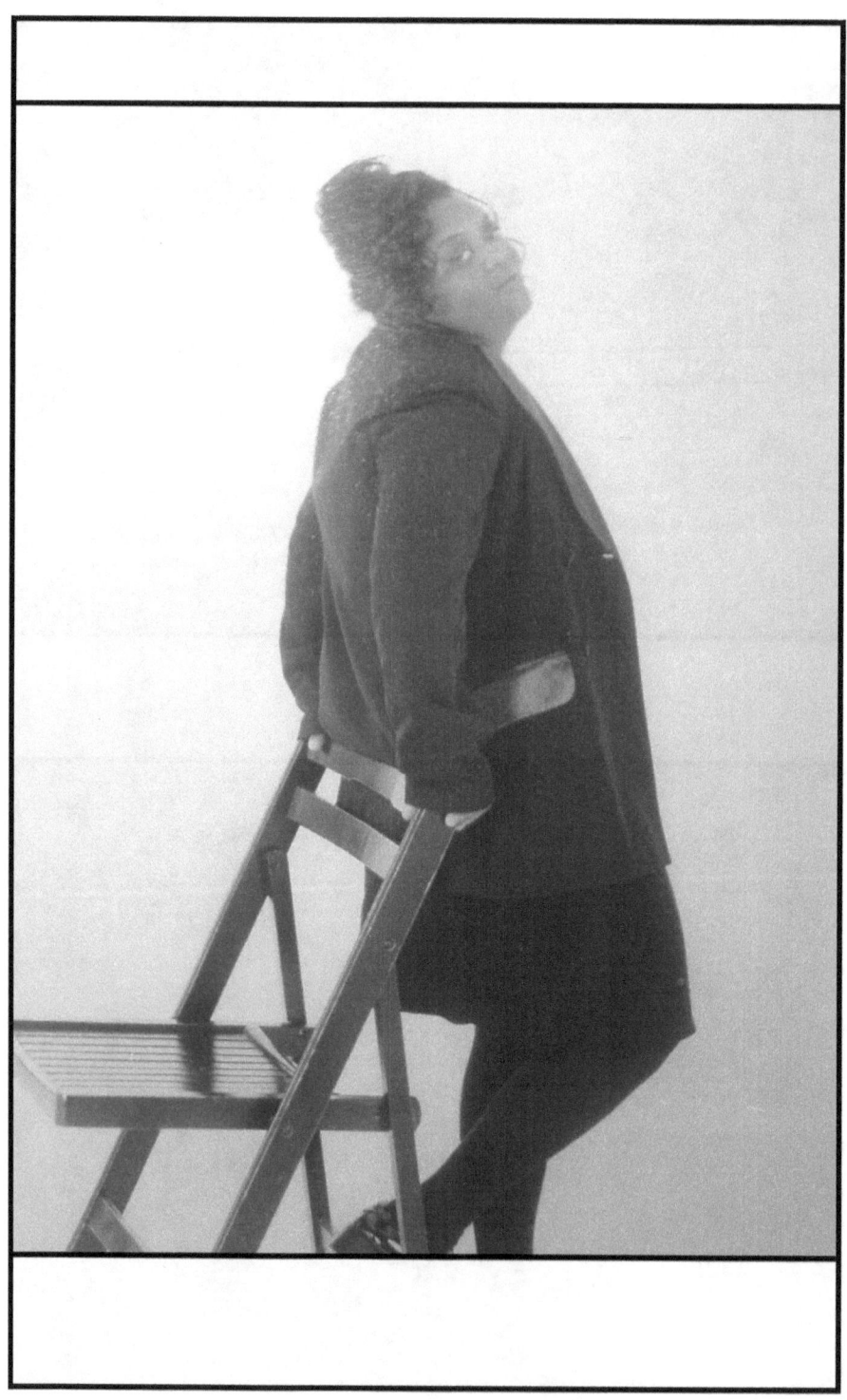

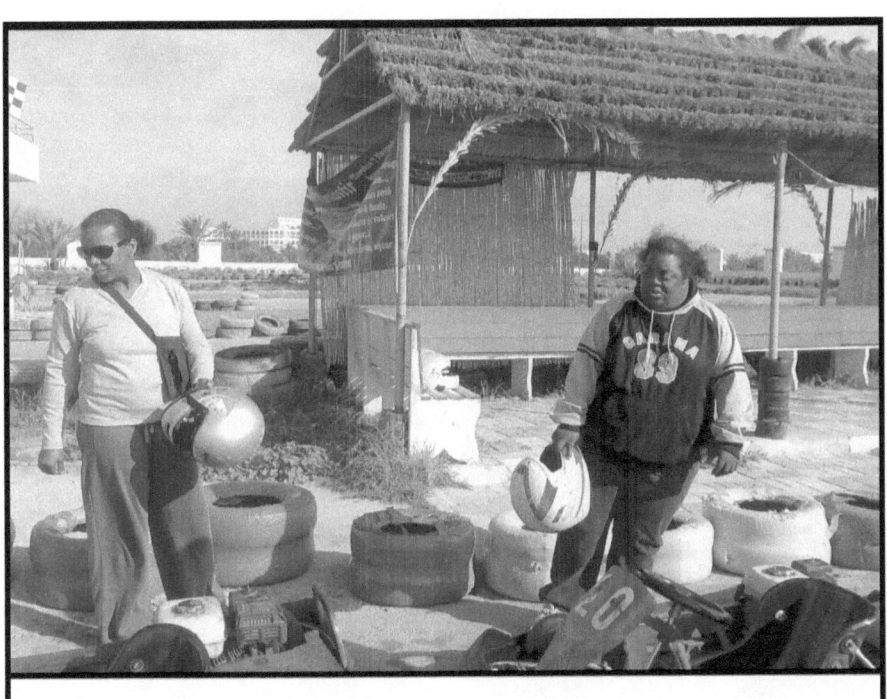

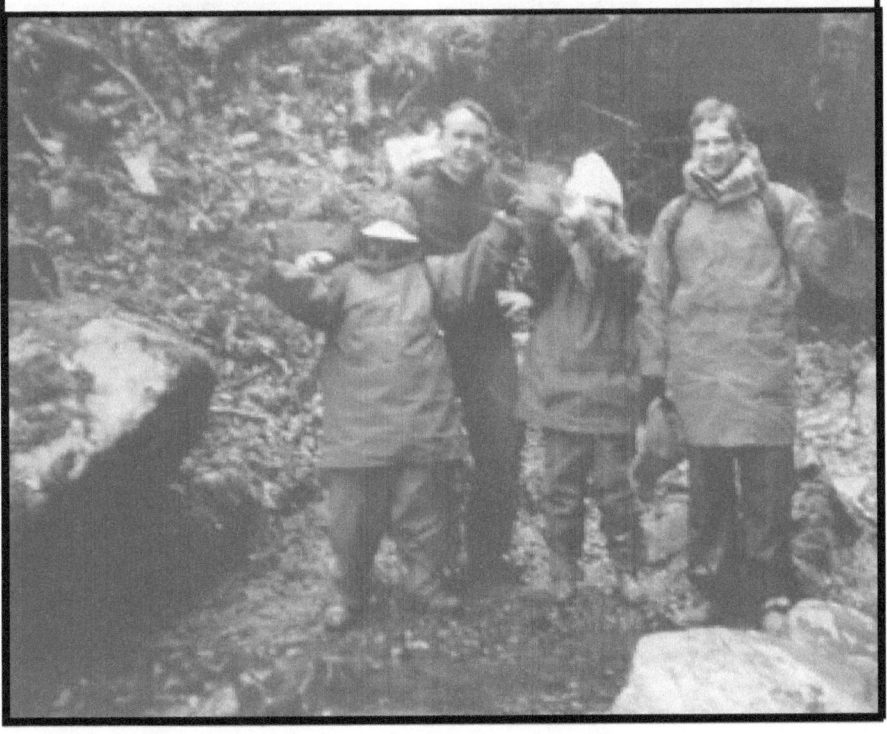

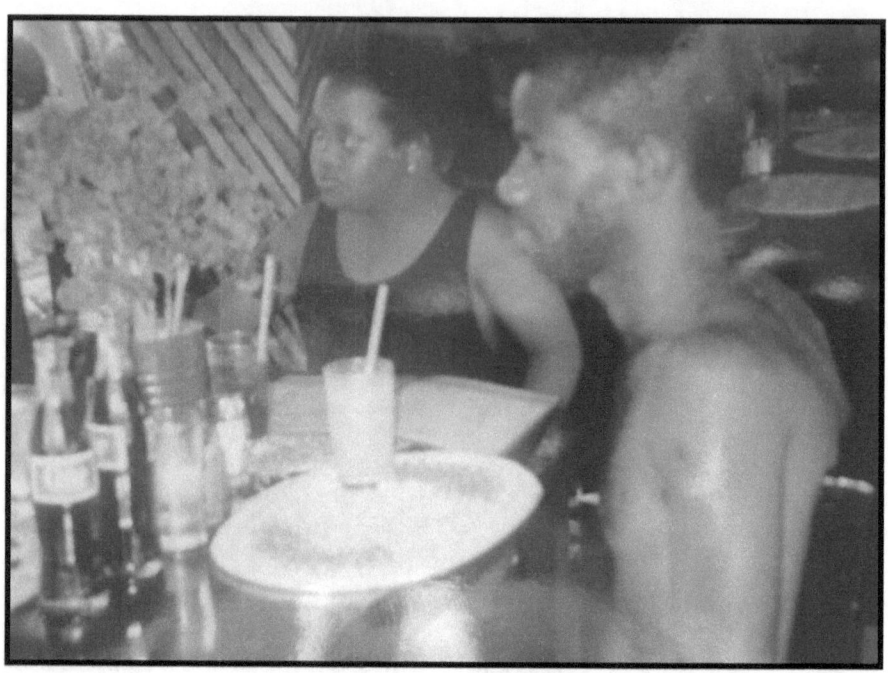

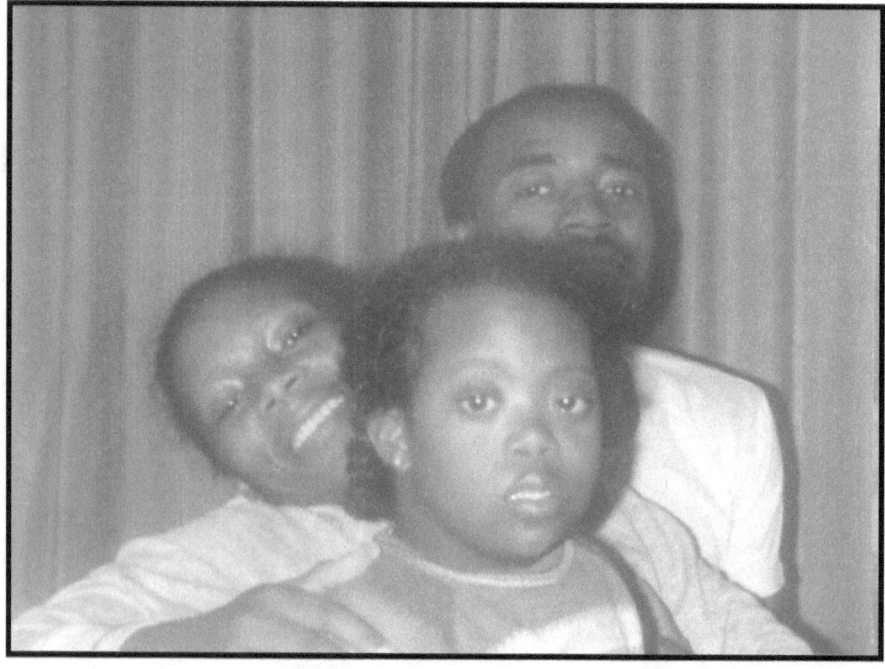

Kaye's Art Work

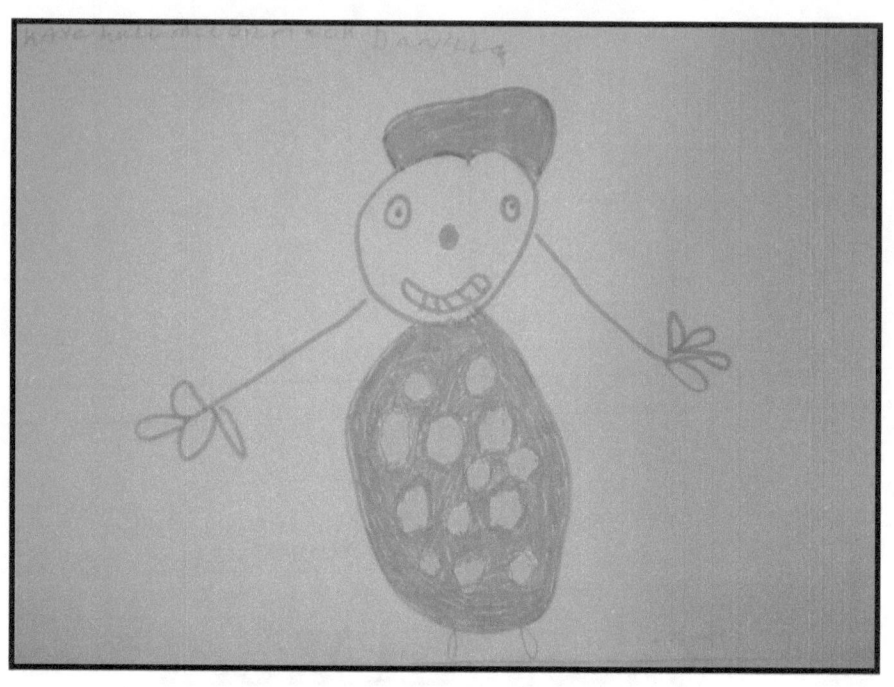

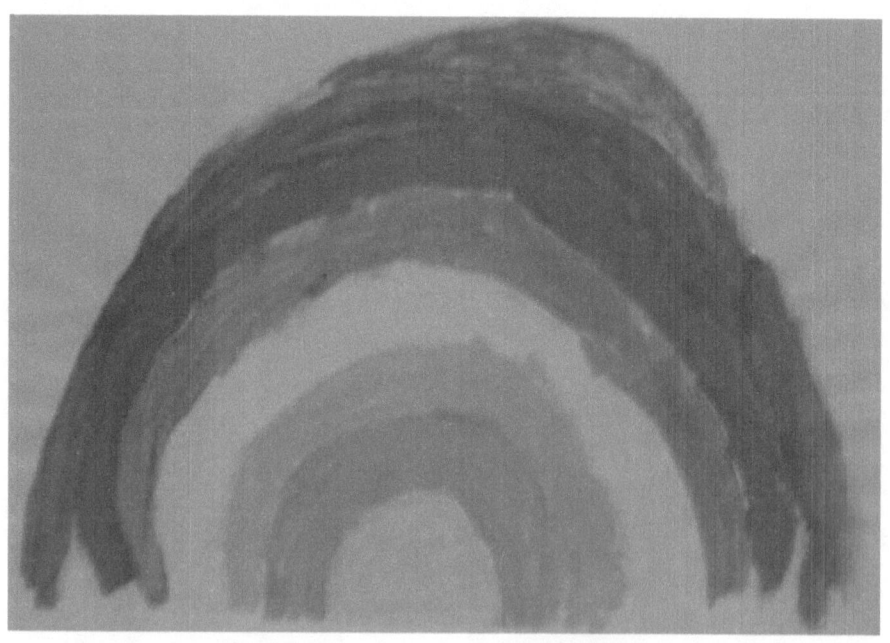

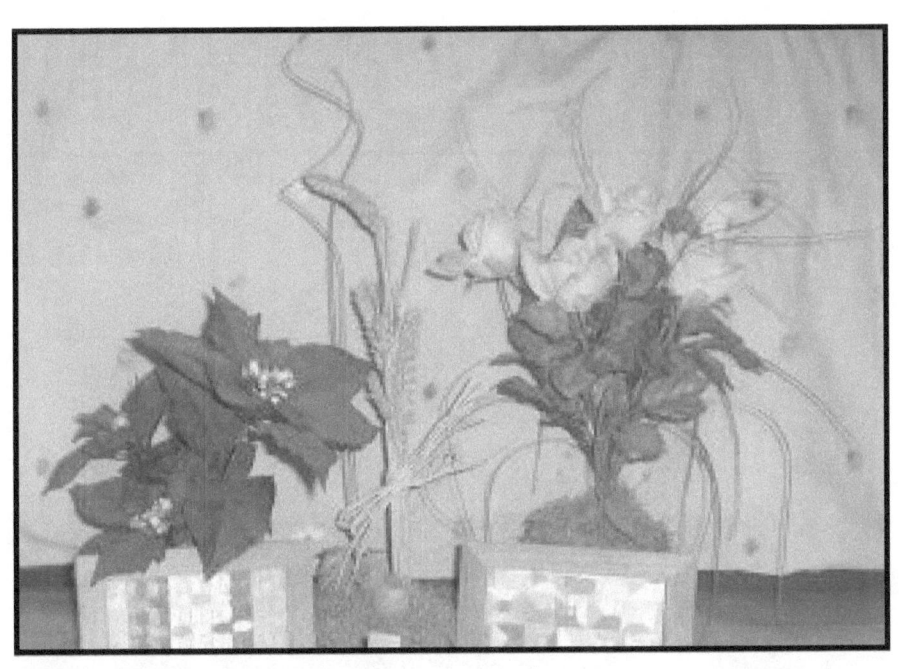

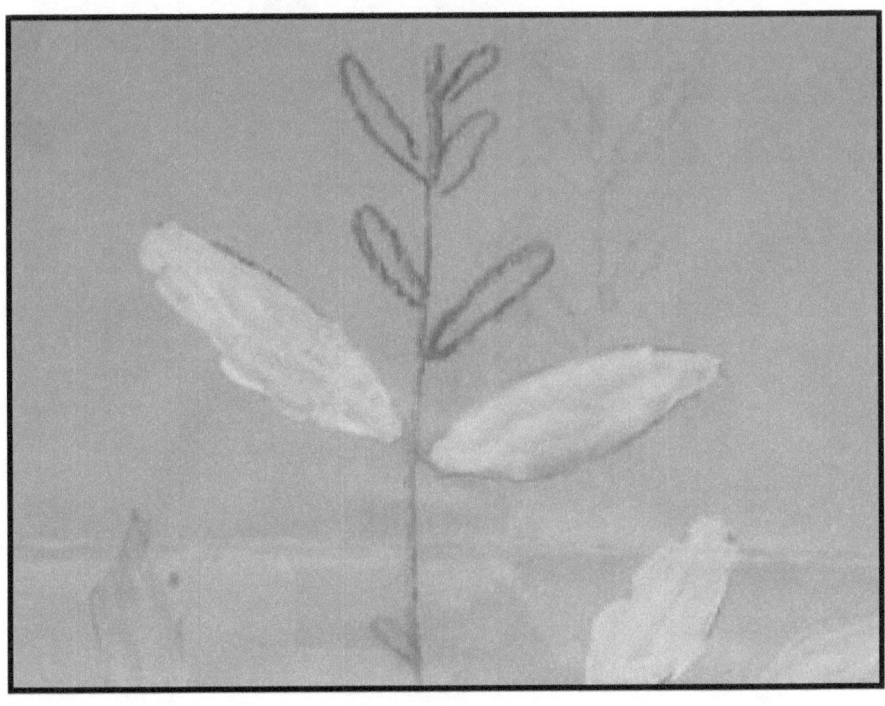

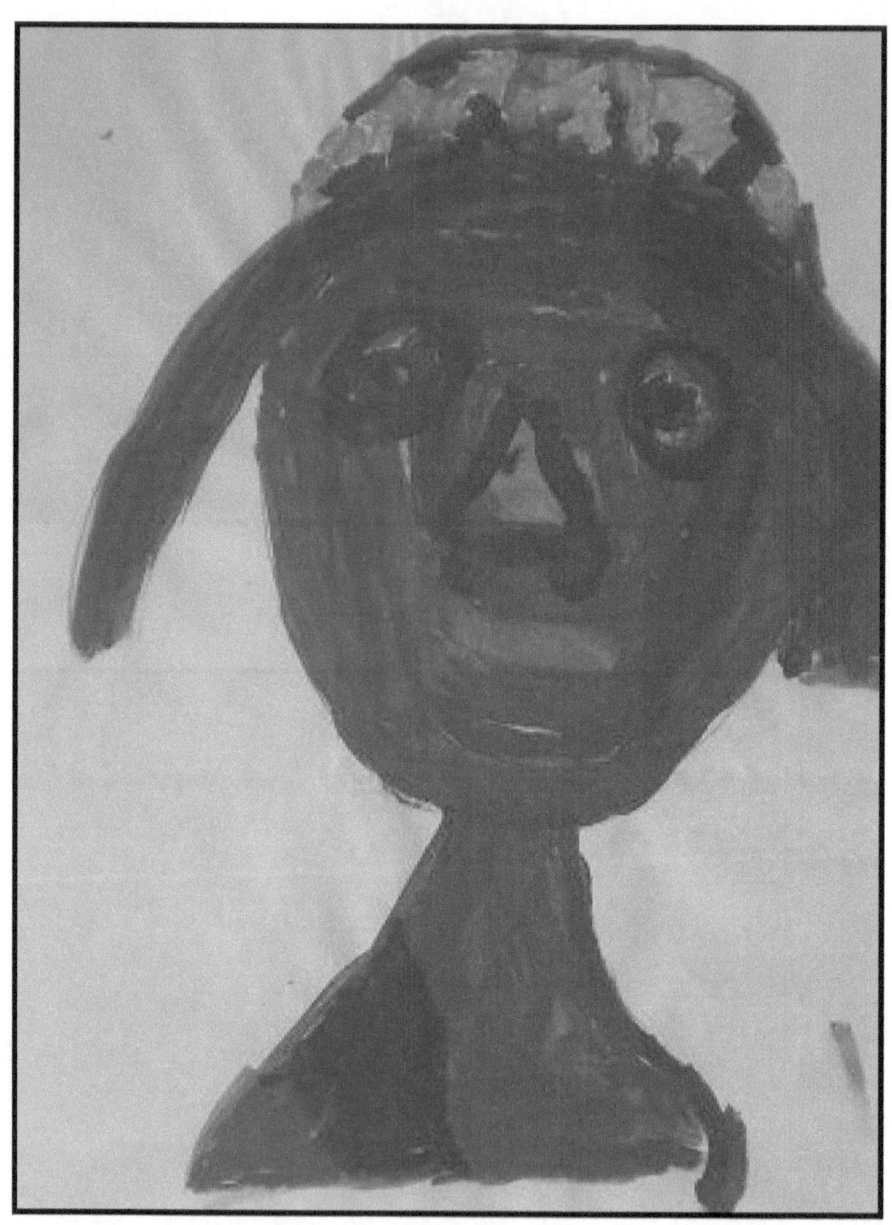

My Memories of Kaye

What I like most about the book.

What I like least about the book.

www.ingramcontent.com/pod-product-compliance
Lightning Source LLC
Chambersburg PA
CBHW031239280526
45784CB00004B/1644